UNVEILING THE HMR PROGRAM

A COMPREHENSIVE GUIDE TO HEALTH

MANAGEMENT RESOURCES

KATE .P

Contents

CHAPTER ONE

INTRODUCTION

The HMR (Health Management Resources) program is a comprehensive weight-loss and lifestyle modification initiative created to support people in improving their general health and achieving long-term weight management. The program, which was created by HMR Weight Management Services Corp., helps people lose weight by combining organized meal replacements, behavioral support, nutrition education, and physical activity.

The foundation of the HMR program is the idea of cutting calories by using portion-controlled meal replacements, like bars, soups, shakes, and meals that are carefully made to support weight loss while offering a balanced diet. These meal replacements make it simpler for users to follow a lower-calorie diet and accomplish long-term weight loss by streamlining portion control and calorie counting.

The HMR program offers meal replacements along with extensive support and direction to assist participants in adopting healthier lifestyle choices. This assistance could take the form of internet resources, individual counseling, group coaching sessions, peer support from those going through a similar weight reduction journey, and more.

The HMR program places a strong emphasis on the value of consistent exercise combined with dietary modifications to support weight loss and enhance general fitness. With planned exercise programs that are customized to each participant's goals and skills, such as walking, strength training, and cardiovascular workouts, participants are encouraged to progressively raise their activity levels.

All things considered, the HMR program offers a methodical and scientifically supported approach to weight management, giving people the instruments, assets, and encouragement they require to attain long-term, sustainable weight loss, enhance their health, and take up healthier lifestyle choices.

An outline of the HMR initiative

Meal replacements, behavioral support, and lifestyle interventions are all included in the HMR (Health Management Resources) program to assist people lose weight sustainably and enhance their general health. An outline of the main elements of the HMR program is provided below:

Structured Meal Replacements: To support weight loss and offer balanced nutrition, the HMR program makes use of portion-controlled meal replacements, such as shakes, entrees, soups, and bars. These meal replacements make it simpler for users to follow a lower-calorie diet and meet their weight loss objectives by streamlining portion control and calorie counting.

Nutrition Education: To assist participants in developing lifetime eating habits, understanding the concepts of balanced nutrition, and making healthier food choices, they provide them with nutrition education and assistance. This instruction supports long-term weight management by covering topics such as macronutrients, portion sizes, reading labels, and meal planning.

Support for Behavior: The HMR program places a strong emphasis on the necessity of changing behavior in order to successfully lose and maintain weight. In order to assist participants overcome obstacles, control cravings, and adopt healthy lifestyle behaviors, trained professionals such as registered dietitians, behavioral health coaches, and certified health educators offer support and direction.

Physical Activity: As it enhances weight loss, increases fitness levels, and promotes general health, regular physical activity is an essential component of the HMR program. Individualized aerobic and resistance exercise regimens, such as walking, running, cycling, strength training, and other activities, are recommended for participants to include in their daily routine.

Friendly Community: Individuals might find a friendly group of peers who are also trying to lose weight. Participants can stay involved and dedicated to their goals with the help of online forums, social support networks, and group coaching sessions, which offer accountability, motivation, and encouragement.

Medical monitoring: For people with specific medical issues or special nutritional needs, the HMR program may offer physician monitoring and supervision. Physicians, nurses, and registered dietitians are among the healthcare experts who collaborate closely with participants to guarantee safe and efficient weight loss results.

Gradual Transition from Meal Replacements to Real Food: As program members advance, they make a gradual switch from meal replacements to real food, emphasizing portion management, well-balanced diets, and wholesome eating practices. This methodical shift assists people in creating long-lasting lifestyle adjustments that promote long-term weight control and general wellbeing.

All things considered, the HMR program offers a methodical, scientifically supported strategy to weight management, giving participants the instruments, assets, and encouragement they require to reach their weight reduction objectives, enhance their well-being, and create long-lasting, healthier lifestyle choices.

Objectives and aims of the HMR initiative

The HMR (Health Management Resources) program's main aims are to help people lose weight in a sustainable way, enhance their general health, and provide them the tools they need to start living better lives. The HMR program's main aims and objectives are as follows:

Encourage Weight Loss: Helping people lose a large and long-lasting amount of weight is the main objective of the HMR program. The program's objectives are to help participants build a calorie deficit so that they can lose weight gradually and consistently over time. It does this by offering organized meal replacements, calorie-controlled eating regimens, and behavioral support.

Enhance Health Outcomes: The HMR program prioritizes enhancing general health outcomes in addition to weight loss. This includes lowering the risk factors connected to diseases like type 2 diabetes, hypertension, high cholesterol, and cardiovascular disease. The program seeks to enhance metabolic health and lower the prevalence of chronic diseases by encouraging a balanced diet, frequent exercise, and lifestyle changes.

Create and Maintain Healthy Lifestyle Habits: The goal of the HMR program is to enable people to create and preserve healthy lifestyle habits that promote long-term weight management and general wellbeing. Through behavioral coaching, support groups, and nutrition instruction, participants learn how to manage cravings, stay active, make better food choices, and get beyond obstacles in their path.

Boost Self-Efficacy: The program aims to boost participants' self-efficacy, or their confidence in their capacity to reach their health and weight reduction objectives. The program helps people develop confidence in their ability to make healthy changes and succeed in their weight reduction journey by offering information, support, and encouragement.

Encourage Sustainability: One of the main goals of the HMR program is to promote sustainability, which highlights the need of making long-term lifestyle adjustments. The program focuses on developing sustainable eating patterns, exercise routines, and behavior improvements that promote continuing weight management and general health rather than providing fast fixes or fad diets.

Establish a Supportive atmosphere: The goal of the HMR program is to establish an inclusive, supportive atmosphere where people are inspired, motivated, and empowered to make positive changes. Along their weight loss journey, members can interact with others, share their stories, and receive encouragement through group coaching sessions, online forums, and social support networks.

Customize treatment: The HMR program acknowledges the value of individualized support and personalized treatment in addition to adhering to a set framework. In order to customize the program to each participant's specific needs, preferences, and goals, healthcare professionals collaborate closely with them to assess their individual demands.

The HMR program strives to assist people in achieving long-term weight loss, enhancing their general health, and embracing better lifestyle choices that enhance their quality of life and long-term well-being by aligning with these goals and objectives.

Recognizing the Elements of the HMR Program

A number of essential elements make up the HMR (Health Management Resources) program, which is intended to help people lose weight, enhance their health, and encourage long-term lifestyle modifications. An outline of the key elements of the HMR program is provided below:

Substitute Meals:

Shakes, dinners, soups, and bars are just a few of the portion-controlled meal replacements that HMR offers in place of typical meals and snacks. These meal replacements are designed to help reduce calories and promote weight loss while maintaining a nutritional balance. They make it simpler for participants to follow a low-calorie diet by streamlining portion control and calorie counting.

Organized Nutrition Program:

The HMR program provides an organized diet plan that includes fruits, vegetables, and other nutrient-dense, low-calorie items along with meal replacements. The participants adhere to a specified eating plan that specifies the quantity of meal replacements to be consumed daily as well as suggestions for extra foods to guarantee a well-balanced diet.

Education on Nutrition:

In order to assist participants make better food choices, comprehend the concepts of balanced nutrition, and form dietary habits for the rest of their lives, they receive thorough nutrition education and counseling. Meal planning, portion control, label reading, dining out techniques, and social scenario management are just a few of the subjects covered in this instruction.

Behavioral Assistance:

A key element of the HMR program is behavioral support, which focuses on assisting participants in acquiring the knowledge and techniques necessary to modify their behavior in a way that will last. Individual counseling, group coaching sessions, and online tools are offered by qualified professionals—registered dietitians, behavioral health coaches, and certified health educators, among others—to assist participants in conquering obstacles, controlling cravings, and embracing healthy living practices.

CHAPTER TWO

Exercise:

As part of the HMR program, regular physical activity is advised to increase fitness levels, aid in weight loss, and support general health. Individualized aerobic and resistance exercise regimens, such as walking, running, cycling, strength training, and other activities, are recommended for participants to include in their daily routine.

a Community of Support:

Access to a peer support network of people who are also trying to lose weight is available to participants. Along their weight reduction journey, individuals can interact with others, exchange stories, and get accountability, motivation, and encouragement through group coaching sessions, online forums, social support networks, and local events.

Medical Supervision:

For those who have particular medical issues or special nutritional demands, the HMR program may include physician observation and supervision. Healthcare providers, such as doctors, nurses, and registered dietitians, collaborate closely with participants to monitor progress, manage any potential difficulties or health issues, and ensure safe and effective weight reduction outcomes.

In general, the HMR program offers a thorough approach to weight control and lifestyle modification by combining meal replacements, nutrition education, behavioral support, physical exercise, and community involvement. The program's goal is to assist participants in achieving long-term weight loss, enhancing their general health, and forming lifelong healthier behaviors by addressing various aspects of health and wellness.

The HMR Science

The HMR (Health Management Resources) program is based on evidence-based weight management and general health improvement practices that are supported by scientific principles. An outline of the science underlying the HMR program is provided below:

Cutting Calories to Lose Weight:

Calorie restriction is the cornerstone of the HMR program and is necessary to achieve weight loss. Through the substitution of portion-controlled meal replacements for traditional meals, participants can efficiently lower their caloric intake while maintaining nutrient intake. Calorie restriction is a critical component of successful weight loss and weight management, as numerous studies have shown.

Effectiveness of Meal Replacement:

Meal replacements, like those included in the HMR program, have been demonstrated in studies to be useful tools for weight loss. Meal replacements help people lose weight by offering portion control, calorie restriction, and balanced nutrition. They also make it simpler for people to follow low-calorie diet plans. Meal replacements have been shown in studies to be more effective in promoting weight loss than conventional low-calorie diets.

Behavioral Techniques:

The HMR program uses support and behavioral tactics to assist participants in changing their lifestyles in a sustainable way. Goal-setting, self-monitoring, problem-solving, and social support are examples of behavioral strategies that work well for encouraging people to follow diet and exercise regimens, control cravings, and get past obstacles in their path.

Education on Nutrition:

A fundamental element of the HMR program is nutrition education, which gives participants the information and abilities to choose better foods and develop balanced eating routines. Studies have indicated that nutrition education initiatives can result in healthier eating habits, wiser selections of foods, and successful long-term weight management.

Exercise:

Frequent exercise is crucial to the HMR program since it increases fitness, aids in weight loss, and improves general health. There are several advantages to exercise, such as higher energy expenditure, better metabolism, better cardiovascular health, and decreased stress. Research has indicated that when diet and exercise are combined, weight loss is higher and weight maintenance is better than when diet is done alone.

Community Assistance:

The HMR program places a strong emphasis on the value of community involvement and social support in assisting with weight loss and lifestyle modifications. Studies have indicated that social support networks, encompassing peer support groups, online forums, and group coaching sessions, can improve health behavior adherence, accountability, and motivation. Individuals who have social support are more likely to reach their long-term weight loss objectives and keep up their progress.

Practices Based on Evidence:

The HMR approach is based on evidence-based practice, which includes suggestions from experts in the disciplines of weight management, obesity, and nutrition, as well as clinical guidelines and research findings. The most recent research findings and industry best practices are used to continuously assess and improve the program's interventions and components.

The HMR program's efficacy in encouraging weight reduction, enhancing health outcomes, and assisting people in adopting healthier lifestyle choices for long-term success is generally supported by the science behind it. Through the use of evidence-based tactics and treatments, the HMR program seeks to enable participants to meet their weight loss objectives and sustain their progress over time.

Options for HMR Programs

A variety of solutions are available through the Health Management Resources (HMR) program to suit a range of interests, objectives, and lifestyles. The following are a few of the various program options:

Within-Clinic Intervention:

The in-clinic program is run in a clinically monitored environment, like a medical clinic or weight management program housed in a hospital. Behavioral health specialists, doctors, and registered dietitians are among the healthcare professionals who provide the participants with individualized support and guidance. Weekly or biweekly appointments, group coaching sessions, medical monitoring, and access to extra services and resources are all possible components of the in-clinic program.

Program for at-home use:

For those who would rather take part in the HMR program virtually from the comfort of their own home, there is an at-home program.

Through online forums, phone or email support, instructional materials, virtual coaching sessions, and online forums, participants receive support and direction. With the flexibility and convenience of the at-home program, participants can follow the HMR program on their own timetable and at their own pace.

Program Without Decisions:

The Decision-Free program is an intense, highly controlled solution for people who would rather utilize meal replacements entirely and wish to lose weight quickly. For a set amount of time usually 12 weeks participants only eat HMR meal replacements, such as smoothies, dinners, soups, and bars. This method makes it easier to stick to a low-calorie diet and lose a considerable amount of weight since it removes the need for decision-making around meal selections and portion sizes.

Program for Healthful Solutions:

A more progressive approach to weight loss is provided by the Healthy Solutions program, which combines meal replacements with extra dietary options. For some meals and snacks, participants use HMR meal replacements, which are augmented with low-calorie items such as fruits, vegetables, lean meats, and other foods. The Healthy Solutions program encourages healthy eating and weight loss while offering flexibility and variety.

HMR at Household Kits:

HMR at Home kits are easy-to-use starter kits that come with everything you need to get started with the program, such as extra support materials, a program manual, and a range of meal replacements. These kits are intended for people who would rather follow the program on their own and might not have access to coaching or support from a coach in person.

Medical Oversight:

Medical monitoring and management for those with certain medical issues or unique dietary needs may be included in some HMR program alternatives. Medical personnel, including doctors, nurses, and registered dietitians, conduct health exams, provide medical monitoring, and customize the program to each patient's needs and goals.

All things considered, the HMR program provides a variety of choices to suit various tastes, lifestyles, and weight reduction objectives. Every participant's preference can be accommodated by an HMR program option, be it rapid weight loss, remote coaching, in-person support, or a more progressive approach.

Benefits and Things to Think About

The Health Management Resources (HMR) program has several benefits for people who want to get healthy, shed some pounds, and change their lifestyle. But, there are additional factors to take into account while determining whether the program is appropriate for you. Below is a summary of the benefits and things to think about related to the HMR program:

Benefits

planned Approach: With meal replacements and extensive support to make portion management and calorie tracking easier, the HMR program offers a planned and simple-to-follow approach to weight loss.

Effective Weight Loss: Studies have demonstrated that the HMR program can result in notable and long-lasting weight loss, with individuals often losing more weight than they would on a conventional low-calorie diet.

Convenient Meal Replacements: Because HMR meal replacements are lightweight and portable, individuals can easily adhere to their diet plan when traveling or on the go.

Nutritionally Balanced: HMR meal replacements are designed to offer vital nutrients and support weight loss in a balanced manner. While cutting calories, participants may be sure they are getting the nutrition they need.

Behavioral assistance: To assist participants in forming healthy habits, overcoming obstacles, and maintaining motivation throughout their weight reduction journey, the HMR program provides behavioral assistance and coaching.

Flexible Program alternatives: The HMR program gives participants the freedom to select the program that best suits their interests and lifestyle. These alternatives include at-home and in-clinic programs, as well as varying degrees of intensity (such Decision-Free and Healthy Solutions).

physician Supervision: To ensure safe and successful weight loss outcomes, certain HMR program choices incorporate physician supervision and monitoring for people with specific medical problems or special dietary demands.

Considering

Cost: Meal replacements, coaching sessions, and training materials may have up-front charges associated with the HMR program. It is important for participants to think about the cost and whether it fits within their budget.

Meal Replacement Dependency: Although HMR meal replacements can make losing weight easier, some people may find it difficult to go back to eating regular meals after using them for a long time. Creating plans for continuing weight loss and good eating after the program is crucial.

Possible Side Effects: During the first stages of calorie restriction, individuals may feel side effects including hunger, exhaustion, or stomach pain, as is the case with any weight loss program. It's critical to pay attention to your body, drink plenty of water, and, if necessary, seek medical assistance.

Adherence and Commitment: Participants' dedication to adhering to the recommended meal plan and program parameters is essential to the HMR program's success. Achieving the best outcomes requires consistency and devotion to the program.

Individual Variation: Depending on a person's metabolism, degree of exercise, medical background, and program adherence, the HMR program's efficacy may differ. It's critical to have patience and realistic expectations when it comes to weight loss.

All things considered, the HMR program provides an organized, empirically supported method of managing weight, with benefits including efficient weight loss, ease of use, and all-encompassing assistance. People who are thinking about the program should be aware of potential drawbacks, though, include expense, the requirement for long-term adherence to sustain results, and dependency on meal replacements. When deciding if the HMR program is right for them, people can make an informed choice by speaking with a certified dietitian or healthcare expert.

Meal Planning and Recipes

A key component of the Health Management Resources (HMR) program is meal planning, which assists participants in adhering to their calorie targets, guaranteeing nutritional balance, and preserving diet diversity. To help you get started, consider the following meal planning advice and HMR-friendly recipes:

Advice for Organizing Meals:

Include HMR Meal Replacements: To guarantee portion control and well-balanced nutrition, include HMR meal replacements in your meal plan. Examples include shakes, dinners, soups, and bars.

Include Fruits and Vegetables: To boost fiber consumption, encourage satiety, and improve overall nutrition, include a lot of fruits and vegetables in your meals and snacks.

CHAPTER THREE

To increase nutrient consumption, go for a range of colored fruits and vegetables.

Select Lean Proteins: To promote muscle maintenance, satiety, and general health, include lean protein sources in your meals, such as skinless chicken, fish, tofu, eggs, and low-fat dairy products.

Select Whole Grains: To add more fiber and nutrients to your diet, opt for whole grains like quinoa, brown rice, oats, and whole wheat bread or pasta.

Watch Portion Sizes: Make sure you are achieving your calorie targets without sacrificing satisfaction by keeping an eye on serving and portion sizes. To portion food correctly, use food scales, measuring cups, and spoons as needed.

Plan Ahead: Give your weekly meal and snack routine some thought, taking into account your calorie targets, preferences, and schedule. Making healthier food choices throughout the week and maintaining organization can be facilitated by creating a meal plan.

Keep Yourself Hydrated: To maintain general health and stay hydrated, make sure you consume lots of water throughout the day. Try to drink eight to ten glasses of water a day, or more if it's hot outside or you're physically active.

HMR-Compatible Recipes:

Smoothie with HMR Chocolate Shake:

Components:

One HMR Chocolate Shake

half a banana

one cup of spinach

One spoonful of butter made of almonds

Half a cup of unflavored almond milk

Directions: Process all ingredients in a blender until they are smooth. Serve right away.

Skewers of grilled chicken and vegetables:

Components:

4 ounces. sliced chicken breast into pieces

Various veggies, including cherry tomatoes, zucchini, and bell peppers

One tablespoon of olive oil

To taste, add salt and pepper.

Directions: Thread veggies and chicken onto skewers. Apply a thin layer of olive oil and sprinkle with salt and pepper. Vegetables should be soft and chicken thoroughly cooked while grilling over medium heat.

Salad with tuna and white beans:

Components:

3 ounces. drained tuna in a can

half a cup of cooked white beans

one cup of mixed greens for salad

One-third cup balsamic vinaigrette

Instructions: Place salad leaves, white beans, and tuna in a bowl. Add a balsamic vinaigrette drizzle and toss to coat.

Stir-fried vegetables:

Components:

One cup of mixed veggies, including snap peas, broccoli, carrots, and bell peppers

3 ounces. extra-firm cubed tofu

One-third cup low-sodium soy sauce

One tsp of sesame oil

Instructions: In a skillet over medium heat, heat the sesame oil. Cook the tofu until it turns brown. Stir-fry the mixed vegetables with soy sauce until they become soft.

HMR Oatmeal with Apple Cinnamon:

Components:

HMR Multigrain Hot Cereal, 1 package

one and a half diced apples

one-fourth teaspoon of cinnamon

One tablespoon of finely chopped walnuts

Instructions: Follow the directions on the package to prepare HMR Multigrain Hot Cereal. Add chopped walnuts, cinnamon, and diced apple and stir. Warm up and serve.

These are just a few illustrations of HMR-friendly meal ideas to assist you in creating wholesome, well-balanced meals while adhering to the program. You are welcome to alter these recipes to fit your dietary requirements and preferences.

Moving Past HMR

Achieving long-term success, keeping healthy habits, and maintaining weight loss all depend on moving past the HMR (Health Management Resources) program. The following advice can help you move past the HMR program:

Gradual Transition: While you can continue to use some HMR products as needed, gradually switch from HMR meal replacements to whole meals by increasing the amount of real, whole foods in your diet. To begin, substitute a whole food alternative for one meal or snack per day, and then progressively expand as you are comfortable.

Emphasize entire Foods: In your diet, place a strong emphasis on entire, minimally processed foods such fruits, vegetables, whole grains, lean meats, and healthy fats. These satiating, nutrient-dense meals offer a variety of vitamins, minerals, and antioxidants to promote general health.

Portion Control: To prevent overindulging and preserve the proper ratio of calories, pay attention to serving and portion sizes. When portioning out foods, especially high-calorie goods like nuts, oils, and starchy carbohydrates, use measuring cups, spoons, and food scales as needed.

Eating Slowly and Savoring Every Bite: To cultivate mindful eating, pay attention to your body's signals of hunger and fullness. When eating, keep electronics like TVs, phones, and computers out of the way to appreciate your food and avoid overindulging.

Frequent Exercise: Make it a priority to engage in frequent exercise as part of your everyday schedule. To support weight maintenance, raise fitness levels, and improve general health, try combining cardiovascular, strength, and flexibility workouts.

Keep Yourself Hydrated: To maintain general health and stay hydrated, sip lots of water throughout the day. Water facilitates normal bodily system functioning, aids in digestion, and helps control appetite. Try to drink eight to ten glasses of water a day, or more if it's hot outside or you're physically active.

Track Your Progress: Weigh yourself frequently, keep an eye on your measurements, and gauge how you're feeling both emotionally and physically to keep tabs on your progress. Enjoy your victories and practice self-compassion while you work through the adjustment.

Seek Support: To help you stay accountable, inspired, and on track with your health and wellness objectives, keep reaching out to friends, family, or support groups. Assemble a supportive and encouraging circle of people around you.

Exercise Self-Compassion: As you face the difficulties of moving past the HMR program, be gentle to yourself and exercise self-compassion. Acknowledge that challenges and failures are inevitable on the path and concentrate on making progress rather than perfection.

Speak with a Professional: For individualized advice and assistance as you move past the HMR program, think about speaking with a registered dietitian, healthcare provider, or weight loss coach. They may offer customized advice, deal with any issues or difficulties, and assist you in developing a workable strategy for long-term success.

You can successfully continue your weight reduction, health gains, and long-term good lifestyle habits beyond the HMR program by using these tactics and ideas. Recall that attaining long-term success requires self-care, perseverance, and consistency.

CONCLUSION

To sum up, the Health Management Resources (HMR) program provides a methodical and scientifically supported strategy to managing weight and enhancing general health. By means of its all-inclusive elements, which comprise meal replacements, education on nutrition, behavioral support, physical activity, and community involvement, the HMR program enables people to attain long-term weight loss, enhance their health outcomes, and embrace healthier lifestyle practices.

Scientific evidence and clinical research support the program's emphasis on calorie reduction, balanced diet, portion management, and behavior modification, confirming its efficacy in facilitating weight loss and enhancing metabolic health. Furthermore, participants can select the program choice that best suits their goals, tastes, and lifestyle thanks to the flexibility and variety it offers.

After completing the HMR program, maintaining weight reduction and maintaining healthy habits involves a progressive shift toward whole foods, mindful eating, regular exercise, and continued support. Through the integration of these tactics into one's everyday existence and the pursuit of assistance from medical experts, friends, and relatives, people can effectively manage the shift and maintain the advantages of their diligent efforts.

All things considered, the HMR program is a great tool for people who want to lose weight, keep it off, get healthy, and live better, more fulfilling lives. Individuals can achieve long-term success and adopt a healthier lifestyle after the program with dedication, persistence, and support.

THE END